# Sensei Self Development

## Mental Health Chronicles Series

*Exploring Self-Care Practices*

Sensei Paul David

# Copyright Page

Sensei Self Development - Exploring Self-Care Practices,
by Sensei Paul David

Copyright © 2024

All rights reserved.

978-1-77848-337-0
SSD_Journals_Amazon_Paperback Book_Exploring Self-Care Practices

978-1-77848-336-3
SSD_Journals_Amazon_eBook_Exploring Self-Care Practices

978-1-77848-455-1
SSD_Journals_Ingram_Paperback_ Exploring Self-Care Practices

This book is not authorized for free distribution copying.

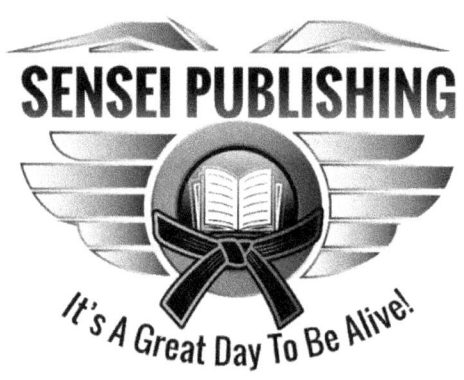

www.senseipublishing.com

@senseipublishing
#senseipublishing

# Get/Share Your FREE SSD Mental Health Chronicles at
# www.senseiselfdevelopment.care

## or

## CLICK HERE

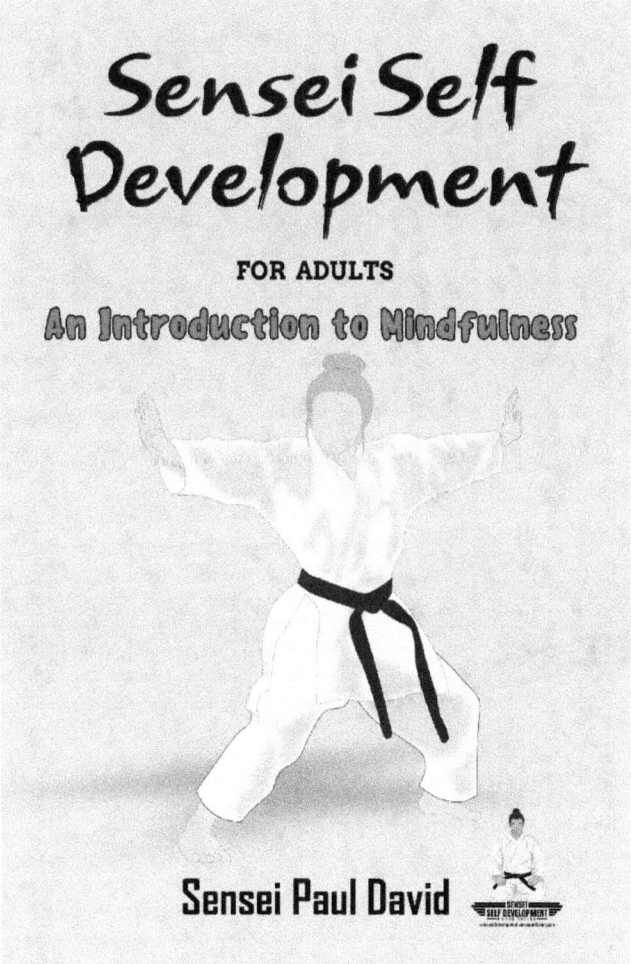

# Check Out The SSD Chronicles Series CLICK HERE

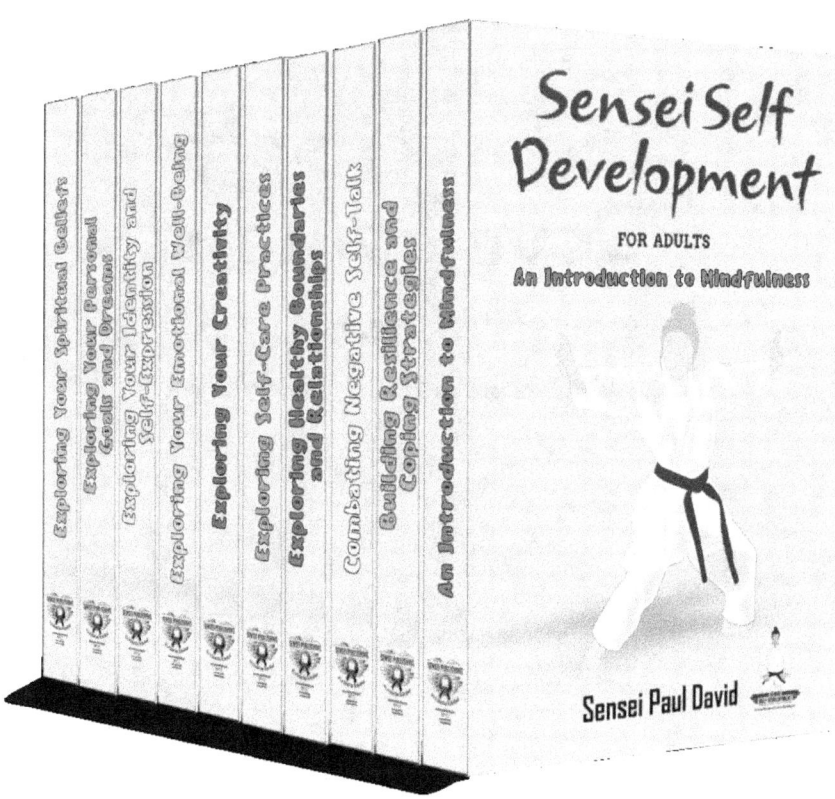

## Dedication

To those who courageously take action towards self-improvement - you are helping to evolve the world for generations to come.

- It's a great day to be alive!

**If Found Please Contact:**

_____


**Reward If Found:**

_____

# MY COMMITMENT

I, _____ commit to writing This Sensei Self Development Journal for at least 10 days in a row, starting: _____

Writing this journal is valuable to me because:

_____
_____
_____
_____
_____

If I finish a minimum of 10 consecutive days of writing in this journal, I will reward myself by:

_____
_____
_____
_____

_____

_____

If I don't finish 10 days of writing this journal, I will promise to:

_____

_____

_____

_____

_____

I will do the following things to ensure that I write in my Sensei Self Development Journal every day:

_____

_____

_____

_____

_____

# Get/Share Your FREE All-Ages Mental Health eBook Now at

www.senseiselfdevelopment.com

## Or CLICK HERE

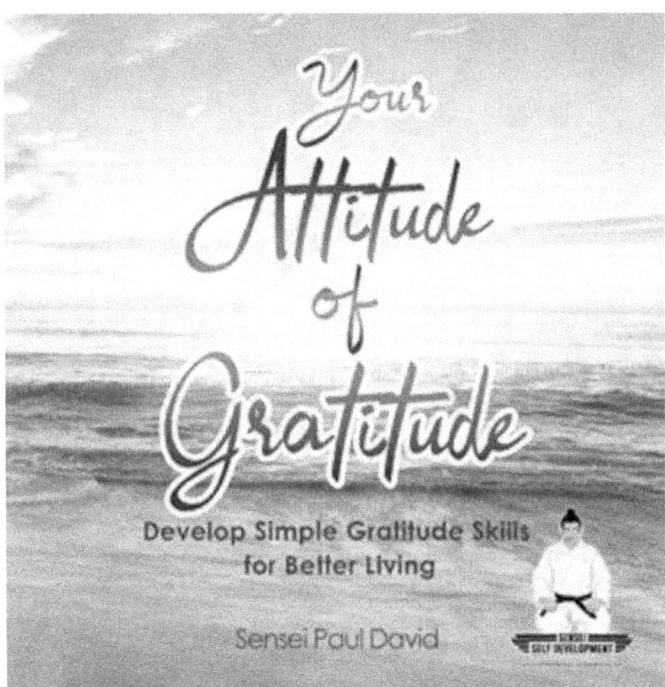

senseiselfdevelopment.com

# Check Out Another Book In The SSD BOOK SERIES:
senseipublishing.com/SSD_SERIES
## CLICK HERE

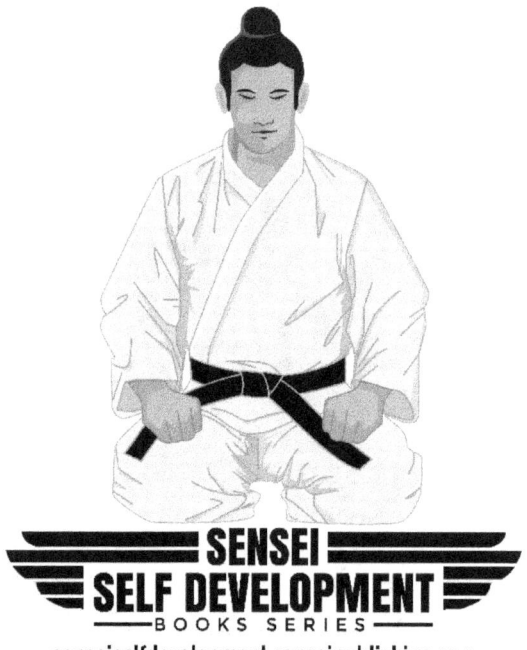

# Join Our Publishing Journey!

If you would like to receive FUTURE FREE BOOKS and get to know us better, please click www.senseipublishing.com and join our newsletter by entering your email address in the pop-up box.

**Follow Our Blog: senseipauldavid.ca**

Follow/Like/Subscribe: Facebook, Instagram, YouTube: @senseipublishing

Scan the QR Code with your phone or tablet
to follow us on social media: Like / Subscribe / Follow

# A Message From The Author:
## Sensei Paul David

Dear Reader,

Welcome to the world of mental health journaling – a sacred space for self-reflection, growth, and healing. Within these pages, you hold the power to uplift your spirit, invigorate your mind, and nourish your goals.

In a world that often moves at blink-and-you'll-miss-it speed, it's crucial to make time for self-care and self-discovery.

Anxiety, stress, and emotional turbulence may have clouded your mind, making it difficult to find clarity and peace within. But fear not! Together, we will navigate the labyrinth of emotions, and experiences, helping to simplify the path to mental well-being.

This journal is not merely a bunch of blank pages awaiting your words. It is your compassionate companion, offering solace and understanding during your unique journey. Here, you are free to unburden yourself, celebrate small and large victories, and confront the challenges that may still linger.

Within the sheltered realm of these pages, there is no judgment, no expectation, and no pressure. Your unique experience and perspective hold immeasurable worth, and your voice deserves to be heard. Whether you choose to fill the lines with eloquence or simply scribble fragments of your thoughts, please remember each entry is a valuable contribution to your growth.

In this sacred space, you are challenged to take off the mask we so often wear in the outside world. It is here that you can be raw, vulnerable, and authentic – allowing your true self to be seen and embraced without reservation. By giving yourself permission to explore the depths of your emotions and confront the shadows that may lurk within, you will discover profound insights and find the healing you seek over time.

As you embark on this journaling journey, I encourage you to embrace the process itself rather than fixate solely on the outcome. Remember, it is not about reaching a certain destination or ticking off boxes on a list of accomplishments. Rather, it is about cultivating self-awareness, fostering self-compassion, and nurturing a sense of curiosity about the intricate workings of your intelligently beautiful mind.

In the quiet moments of reflection, let your pen become a bridge between your inner world and the possibilities that lie ahead. Create a sanctuary for your thoughts, fears, triumphs, and dreams. As you pour your heart onto these pages, allow your words to be a living testament to courage, resilience, and an unwavering commitment to your own well-being.

I am honored to be a part of your journey, and I believe in your ability to navigate the twists and turns with grace and resilience. Remember, you are not alone in this – countless others have walked similar paths, faced similar challenges, and emerged stronger and wiser on the other side. You have the power to reclaim all of your untapped joy, cultivate a positive mindset that serves you, and foster a deep sense of self-love and peaceful confident. – And it will take a worth effort and time.

So, open the first page of this journal with hope, curiosity, and an open heart and open mind. Embrace the transformative power of self-reflection, and allow it to guide you towards a life of greater fulfilment and peace. Each journaling session is an opportunity to not only connect with yourself but also to rekindle the light within that sometimes flickers but never extinguishes.

Remember, the pages you are about to fill are not just a record of your journey but also a testament to your strength, resilience, and indomitable spirit. Cherish this space, invest in yourself, and let your words be an ode to the magnificent journey of becoming whole.

With great respect for your decision to evolve,

Paul

# MY CONVICTION

*Please circle your answers below*

I am DECIDING to be patient with myself and this PROCESS each time I journal toward my improved state of mental well-being

        YES        NO

"The present moment is filled with joy and happiness. If you are attentive, you will see it."

*Thich Nhat Hanh*

# Introduction

In these challenging times, there is no shortage of advice promoting the importance of self-care. We're often encouraged to explore practices like meditation, enjoy soothing baths, and treat ourselves to nurturing products. This advice comes from a place of care, yet it misses the deeper reasons why we fail at self-care.

I frequently meet individuals who earnestly wish to prioritize self-care but find themselves caught in the whirlwind of life's demands. Their own well-being tends to slip to the end of their to-do lists, overshadowed by commitments to work, family, and friends.

Students and young professionals, in particular, face a tough balancing act. The drive to excel in academics, careers, and job applications is formidable. Understandably, by day's end, many are left with little energy to dedicate to their own needs.

Yet, this is exactly what they need.

Abundant research supports the idea that nurturing our minds, bodies, and spirits boosts our effectiveness in everything we do. So, we find ourselves at a crossroads: our mental and physical health are vital for our success, yet our pursuits often leave us with limited time and energy to care for them.

The real solution to making self-care a part of your life isn't just about finding the best sleep or meditation app. It's about changing the way you think about self-care. This book isn't just a list of self-care practices; it's a guide to help you find the ones that suit you best, and more importantly, to help you make them a regular part of your life.

We all know it's easy to feel motivated for a day or two and make big plans. But the real challenge is sticking to those plans. To do that, you need the right mindset and the right strategy.

So let's start this journey. We're going to look at how to adjust our thinking and develop a strategy that works for you, so your self-care becomes a natural, enjoyable part of every day.

## What Is Self-Care?

But before we dive into the nitty gritty, let's see what self-care means.

Self-care is simply about taking steps to look after your health and well-being. It's an open invitation for everyone, and its beauty lies in its flexibility. You can find self-care in the simplicity and cost-free joy of a walk, or in the more involved process of learning a new skill. It encompasses a wide range of activities: it might be saying no to overcommitment, indulging in a purchase that brings you joy, or consciously choosing not to spend.

You can find self-care in a leisurely walk, lending a hand to someone in need, engaging in physical exercise, or immersing yourself in a creative hobby like crafting. It could be organizing things meticulously, such as arranging coins in Ziploc bags, doing some gentle stretching, grooving to disco tunes, or savoring moments of solitude. It might even look like singing your heart out in karaoke, sometimes even on your own, or setting an intention to start a practice like meditation someday.

In essence, self-care is about doing things that bring a sense of peace, fulfillment, and balance to your life, in whatever form that may take for you.

## Figuring Out What Self-Care Means for You

Practicing Jiu-Jitsu has always been a grounding experience for me. Whether it's mastering a new technique, sparring in class, or just drilling the basics, immersing myself in this martial art helps me to focus and find calm amidst life's constant bustle. It's a way for me to step out of the endless stream of thoughts and just be in the moment.

When I'm on the mats, there's no room for distractions or internal monologues. My entire attention is captured by the movements, the strategy of the sport, and the pursuit of improvement. This might be familiar to anyone who's engaged in a physical discipline. While some might find the challenge daunting, I, and others like me, thrive on it.

There's a unique freedom in training without the pressure of a competition or a deadline. I can explore techniques at my own pace, starting when I'm ready and ending when I feel a sense of accomplishment.

Being fully present in each roll, not worrying about anything beyond the mat, is a luxury. The sweat, the focus, the occasional bruises – they're all part of this luxurious experience. Losing myself in the flow of Jiu-Jitsu is one of the most liberating feelings I can imagine.

So Jiu-Jitsu, two times a week, is self-care for me. It might not be for everyone because of the – well – sweat, exhaustion, and tapping out, but it is for me. It gives me confidence, flexibility, and a community (of literal badasses that can choke people out).

Embracing self-care is all about defining it in a way that resonates with your unique needs and desires. With so much advice on self-care out there, it's easy to get caught up in a generic idea of what wellness 'should' look like. But the truth is, only you know what truly nourishes your mind, body, and spirit.

Perhaps for you, unwinding might mean enjoying an episode of your favorite reality TV show after a long day. It might mean seeking support from a therapist or psychiatrist. Or it could be as simple as muting a text chain or a social media thread that's causing you stress.

To discover what self-care means for you, start by paying attention to your own responses. Notice the moments when you feel energized and those when you feel depleted. Look for patterns in your daily life. What activities lift you up? What situations leave you feeling overwhelmed or anxious? Use these insights to start crafting a personal vision of self-care, one that truly fits who you are and what you need.

## Avoid All or Nothing Mindset

Checking for all-or-nothing thinking is a crucial step in developing a healthy approach to self-care. Many people believe they need to completely transform their lifestyle overnight, going from being overwhelmed and sleep-deprived to being a health and fitness guru. This mindset is influenced by the barrage of marketing promising a "new you," but it's far from realistic or helpful.

Recognizing if you're falling into this all-or-nothing trap is the first step toward adopting a more balanced mindset. Once you're aware, you can begin to explore small, manageable changes that fit into your overall life context. It's about gradual improvement, not instant perfection.

As you experiment with these changes, approach the process with curiosity and self-compassion. This mindset is a healthier and more effective alternative to all-or-nothing thinking, often leading to more sustainable and long-lasting changes. Remember, self-care is a journey, not a destination, and small steps can lead to significant improvements in your well-being.

## Avoid These Mindsets

In addition to avoiding all-or-nothing thinking, there are several other mindsets to be mindful of when practicing self-care:

1. Perfectionism: Striving for perfection in self-care routines can be counterproductive. It's important to remember that self-care is about feeling better, not achieving perfection. Embrace imperfection and allow yourself to enjoy self-care activities without the pressure of doing them perfectly.

2. Comparison Trap: Avoid comparing your self-care journey with others. Everyone's needs and circumstances are different. What works for one person might not work for another. Focus on what makes you feel good and what suits your unique lifestyle.

3. Instant Gratification Expectation: Self-care is often a gradual process with cumulative benefits over time. Expecting immediate and dramatic results can lead to disappointment. Patience is key in

recognizing the subtle yet significant changes that self-care brings.

4. Over-Commitment: Taking on too many self-care activities or routines can be overwhelming and unsustainable. It's better to start with a few manageable practices and build upon them gradually.

5. Neglecting Emotional Needs: Focusing solely on physical aspects of self-care like diet and exercise while ignoring emotional well-being is a common oversight. Make sure to balance physical activities with practices that support emotional health, like journaling, therapy, or mindfulness.

6. Guilt-Driven Mindset: Feeling guilty for taking time for self-care is counterproductive. Self-care is a necessity, not a luxury. Remind yourself that caring for your own well-being enables you to be your best for yourself and others.

7. The 'More is Better' Mentality: Believing that more intense or frequent self-care activities will yield better results can lead

to burnout. It's important to find a balance and understand that sometimes, less can be more in self-care.

8. Ignoring Personal Limits: Pushing yourself too hard in the name of self-care, whether it's in exercise, social commitments, or learning new skills, can be detrimental. It's important to recognize and respect your personal boundaries.

9. Discounting Small Victories: Focusing only on big, noticeable changes and overlooking small improvements can be disheartening. Celebrate the small victories and progress, as these are the steps that lead to significant change.

10. Rigidity in Routine: Being too rigid with your self-care routine can make it feel like a chore rather than a nurturing practice. Be flexible and allow yourself to adapt your self-care practices as your life and needs change.

By being aware of these mindsets and actively working to avoid them, you can create a more effective and enjoyable self-care routine that truly benefits your overall health and well-being.

## The Right Mindset

Adopting the right mindset is crucial for effective self-care. Here are several positive mindsets that can enhance your self-care journey:

1. Compassion Over Criticism: Practice being kind and understanding towards yourself. Embrace your flaws and mistakes as part of being human, and treat yourself with the same compassion you would offer a friend.
2. Embracing Individuality: Recognize that self-care is personal and what works for others may not work for you. Celebrate your unique needs and preferences in your self-care routine.
3. Patience and Persistence: Understand that self-care is a continuous process with gradual results. Be patient with yourself and persist in your practices, knowing that

small steps can lead to significant long-term benefits.
4. Balance and Moderation: Aim for a balanced approach to self-care. It's about finding a middle ground that suits your lifestyle and is both enjoyable and sustainable.
5. Emotional Awareness: Pay attention to your emotional needs and incorporate practices that address them, such as journaling, therapy, or mindfulness. Recognize that emotional well-being is as important as physical health.
6. Self-Worth and Prioritization: Believe in the importance of your well-being and prioritize time for self-care without guilt. Acknowledge that taking care of yourself is not a luxury, but a necessity.
7. Celebrating Progress: Acknowledge and celebrate every small step you take in your self-care journey. Recognizing these achievements can be a powerful motivator.
8. Inner Guidance: Trust your intuition and inner guidance when it comes to your self-

care needs. You know yourself best, so trust in your ability to choose what's right for you.
9. Adaptability and Flexibility: Be open to adjusting your self-care practices as your life and needs change. Flexibility in your approach can make self-care more enjoyable and less of a chore.
10. Seeking Balance Between Doing and Being: Recognize the importance of balancing active self-care (like exercise) with passive self-care (like relaxation). Both are equally important in maintaining overall well-being.

By incorporating these positive mindsets into your life, you can build a more effective, enjoyable, and fulfilling self-care practice that nurtures both your physical and mental well-being.

## Trust Yourself

Trusting yourself is a crucial element in the practice of self-care, acting as a guiding principle in choosing what is genuinely beneficial for you. This self-trust means tuning into your own intuition and understanding, recognizing that your path to well-being might look different from someone else's.

In the realm of self-care, a lack of trust in your own judgment can lead you down a path of trial and error with popular methods that might not resonate with your unique needs. This can be an exhausting and disheartening process, where you hop from one trend to another, wondering why these practices aren't yielding the positive results you hear so much about. You might find yourself stuck in routines that don't bring you peace or joy, simply because they are widely recommended.

On the other hand, when you trust your own instincts and knowledge of yourself, you're more likely to identify self-care practices that truly align with your personal needs. For instance, if you find peace in solitary activities like reading or gardening, trusting this preference is key, even if popular advice pushes social activities for relaxation. Similarly, if yoga feels like a burden, and a traditional workout actually feels like Self care to you, then go ahead and get yourself a gym membership.

## The Non-Negotiables

"The Non-Negotiables" in self-care are essential practices that apply universally to all humans, transcending personal preferences. These are fundamental needs that every person requires to maintain their mental and physical health.

1. Adequate Nutrition: Eating a balanced diet with enough nutrients is crucial for everyone. Our bodies need a variety of nutrients to function properly, support the immune system, maintain energy levels, and facilitate overall health. This isn't about specific diet preferences or trends; it's about ensuring that whatever your dietary choices, they provide the necessary nutrients for your body's well-being.

2. **Sufficient Sleep:** Good sleep is a universal requirement. While the exact amount may vary slightly from person to person, the need for quality rest is non-negotiable. Sleep is vital for mental clarity, physical health, emotional regulation, and overall well-being. It's during sleep that the body repairs itself, the brain consolidates memories, and hormones that regulate growth and appetite are released.

3. **Self-Compassion:** Practicing self-compassion is essential for mental health. It involves treating yourself with the same kindness and understanding that you would offer to a good friend. This includes forgiving yourself for mistakes, not being overly critical of yourself, and recognizing that imperfection is part of the human experience.

4. **Physical Activity:** Regular physical activity is essential for maintaining good health. It improves cardiovascular health, strengthens muscles, boosts mental

health, and can improve sleep quality. The form of physical activity can vary – it could be walking, swimming, yoga, or more intense workouts – but the key is that it's consistent and part of your routine.

5. Hydration: Adequate water intake is non-negotiable for maintaining bodily functions. It's essential for digestion, absorption of nutrients, regulation of body temperature, and cognitive functions. Dehydration can lead to a myriad of health issues, both physical and mental.

6. Healthy Relationships: Humans are social creatures, and having healthy relationships is crucial for mental health. This doesn't mean you need a large circle of friends or an active social life. It means having at least a few meaningful connections where there is mutual respect, understanding, and support.

7. Mental Stimulation: Keeping the mind active and engaged is important for everyone. This can be through learning

new things, engaging in challenging activities, or simply indulging in activities that make you think. Mental stimulation is crucial for cognitive health and can be a protective factor against mental decline in later years.

8. Time for Relaxation: Regardless of how busy one might be, finding time to relax and unwind is non-negotiable. This could mean different things for different people, but the underlying necessity is the same – having periods where you are not actively working or stressing, allowing your mind and body to recharge.

These non-negotiables form the foundation of self-care. While individual preferences may dictate how these needs are met, their importance remains universal across all human experiences.

## How to Make it Stick

Benjamin Franklin, well-known for his many achievements, had a practical approach to self-improvement that's still relevant today. He wanted to be a better person, so he made a list of 13 virtues he thought were important, like being organized, honest, and patient.

Instead of trying to work on all these virtues at once, Franklin focused on just one each week. For example, if one week was about being organized, he'd really concentrate on that in everything he did. He kept a simple chart with each virtue and marked it every day he slipped up, like if he was disorganized that day.

This wasn't about being perfect but about getting better bit by bit. Franklin knew it was a long-term effort. He kept cycling through the 13 virtues, spending a week on each. Over time, he found he was making real progress, becoming more like the person he wanted to be.

His story is a great example of how small, consistent efforts can lead to big changes over time. Here's how you can use his method:

1. Choose Your First Self-Care Habit: Start by selecting one self-care activity that feels both important and manageable for

you. This could be something as simple as ensuring you drink enough water each day, taking a short walk in the morning, or setting aside time each evening to read.

2. Define a Clear Objective: Make your goal specific and achievable. For example, if your chosen activity is a morning walk, your goal might be, "I will take a 15-minute walk every morning before breakfast for the next two weeks."

3. Daily Tracking: Like Franklin, who meticulously recorded his progress, maintain a daily log of your activity. This could be in a journal, a calendar, or a digital app. Tracking helps in maintaining accountability and offers a visual representation of your commitment.

4. Weekly Reflections: At the end of each week, take some time to reflect on how the week went. Ask yourself questions like, "How do I feel after implementing this habit?", "What challenges did I face, and how did I overcome them?", and "What

have I learned about myself through this process?"

5. Gradual Expansion: Once your initial self-care habit becomes a natural part of your routine, usually after a few weeks, consider introducing a second habit. Ensure that this new habit is also manageable and meaningful to you.

6. Acknowledge Your Efforts: Recognize and celebrate your commitment to self-care, no matter how small the steps may seem. This could be as simple as acknowledging to yourself that you're doing well, or treating yourself to something special as a reward.

7. Adapt as Needed: Be prepared to modify your routine as you go. If you find a particular habit isn't serving you as expected, it's okay to adjust it or replace it with something more fitting.

By adopting Franklin's focused approach, you can build a self-care routine that is not only manageable but also deeply integrated into your daily life. This method emphasizes patience, consistency, and a gentle progression, allowing you to nurture your well-being one step at a time.

## Is Self-Care Selfish?

Self-care is often misunderstood as selfish, but it's an essential part of maintaining good mental, emotional, and physical health. Think of it like recharging your batteries: when you take time for yourself, you replenish your energy, making you more resilient and better equipped to face life's challenges. It's not just about your well-being; when you're well-cared for, you can care for others more effectively. Constantly putting others first can lead to burnout, frustration, and even resentment. By practicing self-care, you maintain a healthy balance between your needs and those of the people around you.

Self-care also boosts productivity and creativity. When you take breaks and allow yourself some downtime, you come back to your tasks with a more focused and efficient mindset. So, in essence, self-care isn't selfish at all; it's a crucial aspect of living a balanced and fulfilling life, enabling you to be present and effective in all areas.

Selfishness, on the other hand, is all about me, me, me, where the main goal is to gain as much as possible for oneself, sometimes even if it means others lose out. This is quite different from self-care.

Here's a look at how self-care differs from selfishness:

- Self-Care: Prioritizing enough sleep each night.
- Selfish: Oversleeping regularly to dodge responsibilities.
- Self-Care: Taking a break at work to recharge with a healthy meal.
- Selfish: Extending your lunch break beyond allowed limits, neglecting work duties.
- Self-Care: Setting and maintaining healthy personal boundaries.

- Selfish: Consistently refusing to help others without valid reasons.
- Self-Care: Allocating time for relaxation and meditation.
- Selfish: Withdrawing from family and friends, ignoring their needs.
- Self-Care: Buying ingredients to cook a favorite meal.
- Selfish: Using family savings for unnecessary luxury purchases.

## Caution: Dark Playground.

Have you ever found yourself lounging around or playing games, but not actually loving it when you should? I feel that way when I have not earned my free time. If you play games for hours and then try to take a warm bath because you want to practice self-care, you will probably feel shitty.

This is what you can call the Dark Playground. The "Dark Playground" is a concept introduced by Tim Urban, the writer behind the blog "Wait

But Why." It refers to a state of mind where a person procrastinates, engaging in unproductive activities while being fully aware that they are avoiding their important tasks. This state is called a "playground" because it involves activities that are normally enjoyable or relaxing. However, it's termed "dark" because this enjoyment is overshadowed by guilt and stress, knowing that one is procrastinating.

In this state, the procrastinator is not truly relaxed or enjoying the leisure activities because they are burdened by the awareness of what they should be doing. It's a paradoxical situation where the person is neither working nor effectively relaxing, leading to feelings of anxiety and dissatisfaction.

So, you have to be careful your self-care does not get sidetracked into self-indulgence, where you hop from one self-care activity to another.

If you are avoiding your work, you will not feel good doing your self-care activities. What those things are depends on you. It could be related to your job, your education, or your art.

It could even be working out. It could be anything that you need to get done.

But only when you have been productive and not slacking off can you enjoy self-care.

Before We Get Started…

Remember, mindfulness journaling is a personal practice, and these questions are meant to guide and inspire you. Feel free to adapt and modify them to suit your needs and preferences. Explore, reflect, and embrace the opportunity to deepen your self-awareness and cultivate a sense of inner peace.

Date __/__/__: S  M  T  W  Th  F  S

**I feel:**
(please circle)

because _____  because _____  because _____  because _____  because _____

## Today I Am Grateful For
1. _____
2. _____
3. _____

What could help transform today into a remarkable day?

## Reflective Writing
How have my self-care practices changed since exploring this journal?

_____
_____
_____
_____
_____
_____
_____

**Which of the following is NOT considered a self-care practice?**

A) Spending time with loved ones
B) Watching TV for hours
C) Getting enough sleep
D) Practicing mindfulness

All Are Correct - Choose The Response You Feel Is Most Important To Remember

Date ___/___/___ : S  M  T  W  Th  F  S

**I feel:**
(please circle)

because _____ because _____ because _____ because _____ because _____

### Today I Am Grateful For
1. _____
2. _____
3. _____

What could help transform today into a remarkable day?

### Reflective Writing
What have I learned about myself that I didn't know before exploring this journal?

_____
_____
_____
_____
_____
_____
_____

**What is a common issue that can arise from neglecting self-care?**

A) Decreased productivity
B) Improved mental health
C) Increased energy levels
D) Higher self-esteem

All Are Correct - Choose The Response You Feel Is Most Important To Remember

Date ___/___/___ : S  M  T  W  Th  F  S

**I feel:**
(please circle)

😊 because _____
😁 because _____
😋 because _____
😞 because _____
😠 because _____

## Today I Am Grateful For
1. _____
2. _____
3. _____

What could help transform today into a remarkable day?

## Reflective Writing

What are some of the benefits of taking the time to practice self-care?

_____
_____
_____
_____
_____
_____
_____

## Which of the following is an example of physical self-care?

A) Meditating
B) Eating a balanced diet
C) Journaling
D) Setting personal boundaries

All Are Correct - Choose The Response You Feel Is Most Important To Remember

Date ___/___/___ : S  M  T  W  Th  F  S

**I feel:**
(please circle)

because _____  because _____  because _____  because _____  because _____

## Today I Am Grateful For
1. _____
2. _____
3. _____

What could help transform today into a remarkable day?

## Reflective Writing
What are some of the challenges I have faced in trying to prioritize self-care?

_____
_____
_____
_____
_____
_____
_____

**Why is it important to set boundaries for yourself in terms of self-care?**

A) It allows you to prioritize your needs
B) It helps others understand your limitations
C) It can lead to healthier relationships
D) All of the above

All Are Correct - Choose The Response You Feel Is Most Important To Remember

Date ___/___/___ : S  M  T  W  Th  F  S

**I feel:**
(please circle)

because _____  because _____  because _____  because _____  because _____

### Today I Am Grateful For
1. _____
2. _____
3. _____

What could help transform today into a remarkable day?

### Reflective Writing
What have I learned about the importance of self-care in my life?

_____
_____
_____
_____
_____
_____
_____

**Which of the following can be considered an emotional self-care practice?**

A) Taking a relaxing bubble bath
B) Going for a walk in nature
C) Talking to a trusted friend about your feelings
D) Checking emails before bed

All Are Correct - Choose The Response You Feel Is Most Important To Remember

Date ___/___/___ : S  M  T  W  Th  F  S

**I feel:**
(please circle)

because _____  because _____  because _____  because _____  because _____

## Today I Am Grateful For

1. _____
2. _____
3. _____

What could help transform today into a remarkable day?

## Reflective Writing

How have I been able to apply the techniques I have learned from exploring this journal to my daily life?

_____
_____
_____
_____
_____
_____
_____
_____

## How often should you practice self-care?

A) Once a week
B) Only when you feel overwhelmed
C) Daily
D) Once a month

All Are Correct - Choose The Response You Feel Is Most Important To Remember

Date ___/___/___ : S  M  T  W  Th  F  S

**I feel:**
(please circle)

because _____  because _____  because _____  because _____  because _____

### Today I Am Grateful For
1. _____
2. _____
3. _____

What could help transform today into a remarkable day?

### Reflective Writing
How have my relationships with others changed since I have taken the time to practice self-care?

_____
_____
_____
_____
_____
_____
_____

**Which of the following is an example of a spiritual self-care practice?**

A) Going to therapy
B) Writing in a gratitude journal
C) Reading a book for pleasure
D) Attending a worship service

All Are Correct - Choose The Response You Feel Is Most Important To Remember

Date ___/___/___ : S  M  T  W  Th  F  S

**I feel:**
(please circle)

😊 because _____
😁 because _____
😋 because _____
😟 because _____
😠 because _____

## Today I Am Grateful For
1. _____
2. _____
3. _____

What could help transform today into a remarkable day?

### Reflective Writing
What are some of the creative ways I have found to prioritize self-care?

_____
_____
_____
_____
_____
_____
_____

**What is a sign that you may be experiencing burnout and need to focus on self-care?**

A) Feeling guilty for taking time for yourself
B) Difficulty concentrating
C) Feeling energized and motivated
D) Increased self-confidence

All Are Correct - Choose The Response You Feel Is Most Important To Remember

Date ___/___/___ : S M T W Th F S

**I feel:**
(please circle)

😊 because _____
😁 because _____
😋 because _____
😟 because _____
😠 because _____

### Today I Am Grateful For
1. _____
2. _____
3. _____

What could help transform today into a remarkable day?

### Reflective Writing
What have I learned about personal boundaries and how they relate to self-care?

_____
_____
_____
_____
_____
_____
_____

**Which of the following is NOT a benefit of practicing self-care?**

A) Improved physical health
B) Reduced stress and anxiety
C) Increased self-criticism
D) Enhanced overall well-being

All Are Correct - Choose The Response You Feel Is Most Important To Remember

Date ___/___/___ : S  M  T  W  Th  F  S

**I feel:**
(please circle)

😊 because _____
😁 because _____
😋 because _____
😟 because _____
😠 because _____

## Today I Am Grateful For
1. _____
2. _____
3. _____

What could help transform today into a remarkable day?

### Reflective Writing
What have I learned about the importance of self-love and how it relates to self-care?

_____
_____
_____
_____
_____
_____
_____

**How can practicing self-care benefit your relationships?**

A) It can improve communication and empathy
B) It can make you more agreeable and easy-going
C) It can help you avoid conflict
D) It can make you more self-centered and less empathetic

All Are Correct - Choose The Response You Feel Is Most Important To Remember

Date ___/___/___ : S  M  T  W  Th  F  S

**I feel:**
(please circle)

😊 because _____
😁 because _____
😋 because _____
😟 because _____
😠 because _____

### Today I Am Grateful For
1. _____
2. _____
3. _____

What could help transform today into a remarkable day?

## Reflective Writing

What have I learned about the connection between physical health and self-care?

_____
_____
_____
_____
_____
_____
_____

**What is one way to practice self-care while still maintaining a busy schedule?**

A) Skip meals to save time
B) Multitask while completing self-care activities
C) Sacrifice sleep to get more done
D) Prioritize and schedule self-care into your routine

All Are Correct - Choose The Response You Feel Is Most Important To Remember

Date ___/___/___ : S  M  T  W  Th  F  S

I feel:
(please circle)

because _____  because _____  because _____  because _____  because _____

### Today I Am Grateful For
1. _____
2. _____
3. _____

What could help transform today into a remarkable day?

## Reflective Writing
What are some of the ways I have been able to practice self-care when I'm feeling overwhelmed?

_____
_____
_____
_____
_____
_____
_____

**What is a key aspect of practicing self-care?**

A) Doing activities that you dislike but are good for you
B) Copying the self-care practices of others
C) Taking care of others before taking care of yourself
D) Prioritizing activities that bring joy and rejuvenation to you

All Are Correct - Choose The Response You Feel Is Most Important To Remember

Date ___/___/___ : S  M  T  W  Th  F  S

**I feel:**
(please circle)

😊 because _____  😁 because _____  😋 because _____  😞 because _____  😠 because _____

### Today I Am Grateful For
1. _____
2. _____
3. _____

What could help transform today into a remarkable day?

## Reflective Writing
How have my emotions and mental state changed since I have taken the time to practice self-care?

_____
_____
_____
_____
_____
_____
_____
_____

**Which of the following activities is NOT a form of self-care?**

A) Eating a salad
B) Taking a long bubble bath
C) Watching a movie with friends
D) Checking social media for hours

All Are Correct - Choose The Response You Feel Is Most Important To Remember

Date ___/___/___ : S  M  T  W  Th  F  S

**I feel:**
(please circle)

because _____  because _____  because _____  because _____  because _____

### Today I Am Grateful For
1. _____
2. _____
3. _____

What could help transform today into a remarkable day?

## Reflective Writing
What have I learned about the importance of setting aside time for self-care?

_____
_____
_____
_____
_____
_____
_____

**How can practicing self-care positively impact your mental health?**

A) It can reduce symptoms of depression and anxiety
B) It can increase feelings of loneliness and isolation
C) It can lead to overthinking and self-criticism
D) It can cause feelings of guilt and shame

All Are Correct - Choose The Response You Feel Is Most Important To Remember

Date ___/___/___ : S  M  T  W  Th  F  S

**I feel:** 😊 😁 😋 😟 😠
(please circle) because because because because because
___  ___  ___  ___  ___

### Today I Am Grateful For
1. _____
2. _____
3. _____

What could help transform today into a remarkable day?

### Reflective Writing
How have my relationships with myself and others changed since I have taken the time to practice self-care?

_____
_____
_____
_____
_____
_____
_____

**Why is it important to practice self-care when facing challenges or difficult situations?**

A) It can be a coping mechanism to help you deal with stress
B) It is a form of procrastination
C) It demonstrates laziness and lack of productivity
D) It is a way to avoid facing your problems

All Are Correct - Choose The Response You Feel Is Most Important To Remember

As we reach the final pages of this journey through "Positive Mindset," I want to extend my heartfelt thanks to you. Your commitment to exploring positivity and its transformative power is not only commendable but a testament to your desire for personal growth and a richer, more fulfilling life experience.

Remember, the journey towards a positive mindset is ongoing and ever-evolving. Each day presents new opportunities to apply these principles, to learn, and to grow. I encourage you to revisit these pages whenever you need a reminder of your incredible potential to foster positivity and resilience in the face of life's challenges.

As we part ways, I leave you with a quote that has been a guiding star in my journey: "The greatest discovery of any generation is that a human can alter his life by altering his attitude."

– William James.

Thank you for allowing me to be a part of your journey. May your path be filled with light, hope, and endless possibilities. Farewell, and may you carry the spirit of positivity with you, today and always.

With gratitude and best wishes,

Sensei Paul David

# Reflective Writing

# The End

As you close the pages of this mindfulness journal, remember that each word you've written is a step on your journey towards self-awareness and inner peace. Embrace the moments of clarity, the revelations, and even the uncertainties you've encountered along the way. Let this journal be a testament to your growth and a reminder that every day offers a new opportunity to be present, to observe, and to appreciate the simple wonders of life. Carry these lessons forward, and may your path be filled with mindful moments and serene reflections. Until we meet again in these pages, be gentle with yourself and stay anchored in the now.

Mindfulness isn't difficult, we just need to remember to do it.

# Thank You!

If you found this book helpful, I would be grateful if you would **post an honest review on Amazon** so this book can reach other supportive readers like you!

All you need to do is digitally flip to the back and leave your review. Or visit amazon.com/author/senseipauldavid click the correct book cover and click on the blue link next to the yellow stars that say, "customer reviews."

## *As always...*
## *It's a great day to be alive!*

# Get/Share Your FREE SSD Mental Health Chronicles at www.senseiselfdevelopment.care

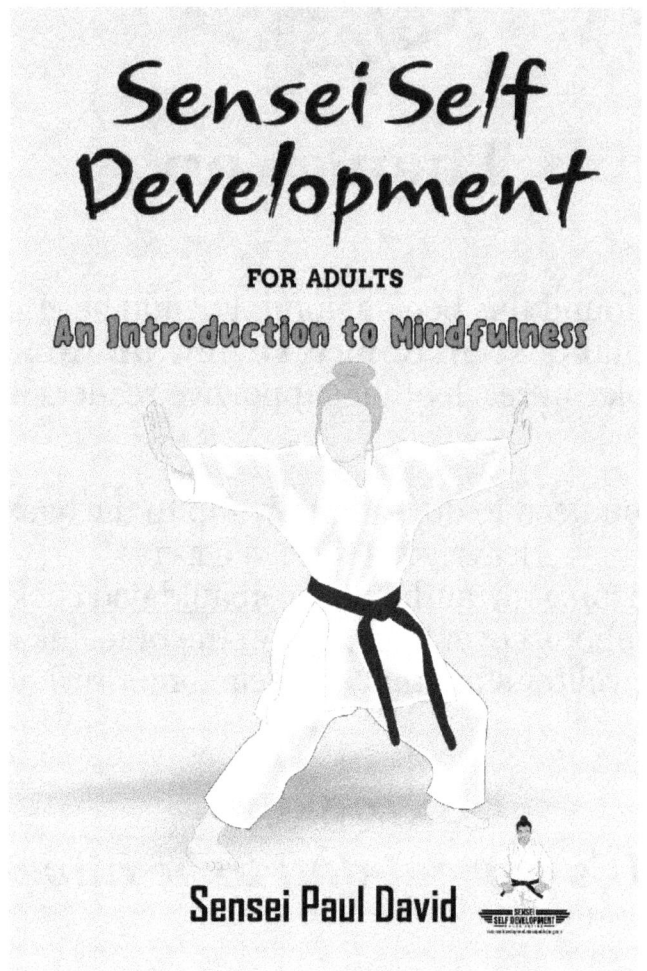

# Check Out The SSD Chronicles Series CLICK HERE

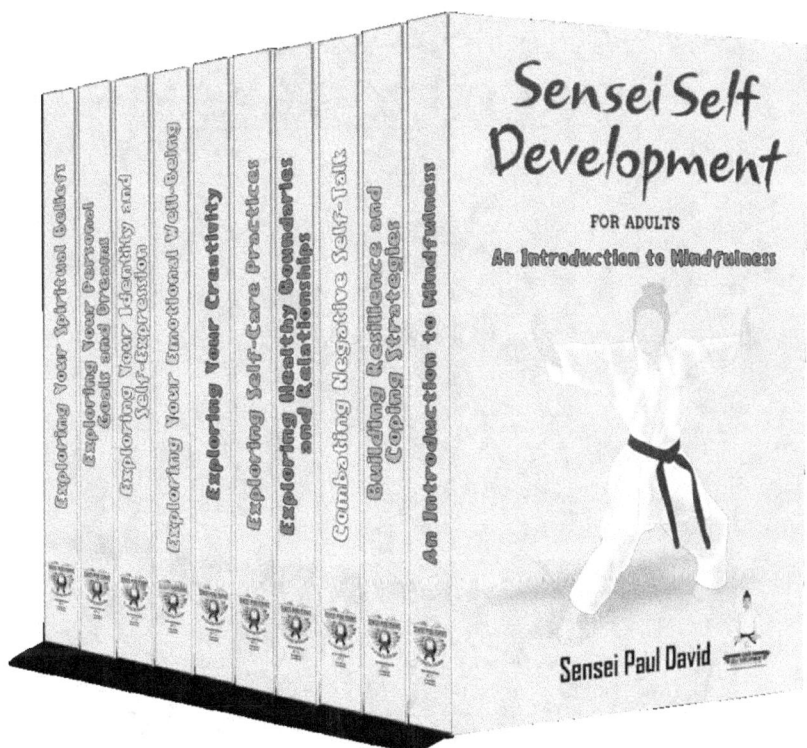

# Get/Share Your FREE All-Ages Mental Health eBook Now at

www.senseiselfdevelopment.com

## Or CLICK HERE

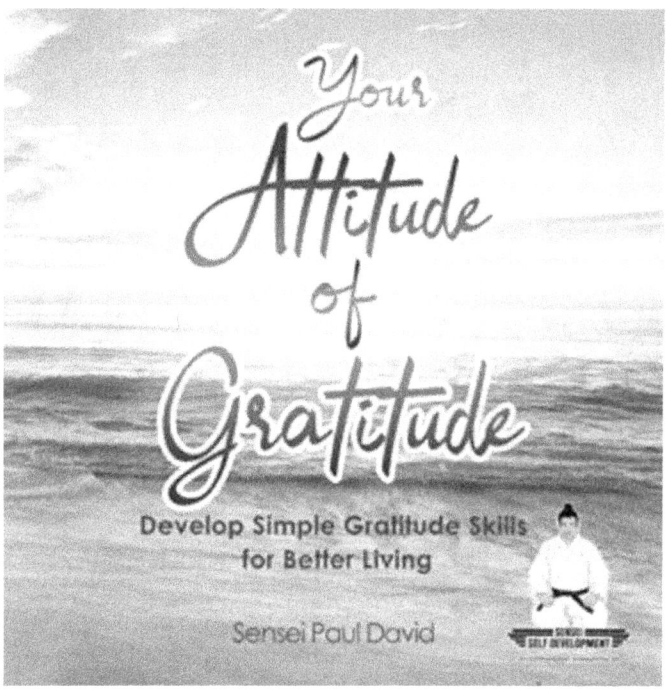

senseiselfdevelopment.com

# Click Another Book In The SSD BOOK SERIES:
senseipublishing.com/SSD_SERIES
## CLICK HERE

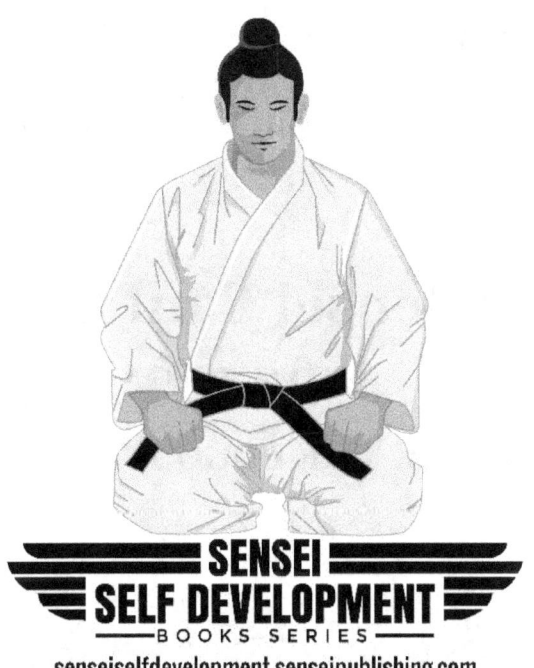

# Join Our Publishing Journey!

If you would like to receive FREE BOOKS, please visit **www.senseipublishing.com**. Join our newsletter by entering your email address in the pop-up box

# Follow Sensei Paul David on Amazon

## CLICK THE LOGO BELOW

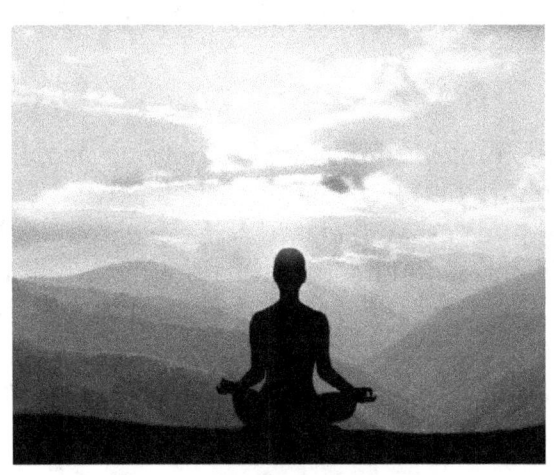

## FREE BONUS!!!
## Experience Over 25 FREE Engaging Guided Meditations!

Prized Skills & Practices for Adults & Kids. Help Restore Deep-Sleep, Lower Stress, Improve Posture, Navigate Uncertainty & More.

Download the Free Insight Timer App and click the link below:
**http://insig.ht/sensei_paul**

# About Sensei Publishing

Sensei Publishing commits itself to helping people of all ages transform into better versions of themselves by providing high-quality and research-based self-development books with an emphasis on mental health and guided meditations. Sensei Publishing offers well-written e-books, audiobooks, paperbacks and online courses that simplify complicated but practical topics in line with its mission to inspire people towards positive transformation.

It's a great day to be alive!

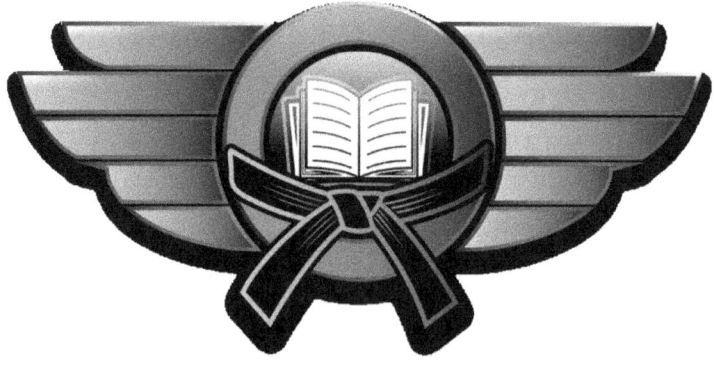

# About the Author

I create simple & transformative eBooks & Guided Meditations for Adults & Children proven to help navigate uncertainty, solve niche problems & bring families closer together.

I'm a former finance project manager, private pilot, jiu-jitsu instructor, musician & former University of Toronto Fitness Trainer. I prefer a science-based approach to focus on these & other areas in my life to stay humble & hungry to evolve. I hope you enjoy my work and I'd love to hear your feedback.

- It's a great day to be alive!

Sensei Paul David

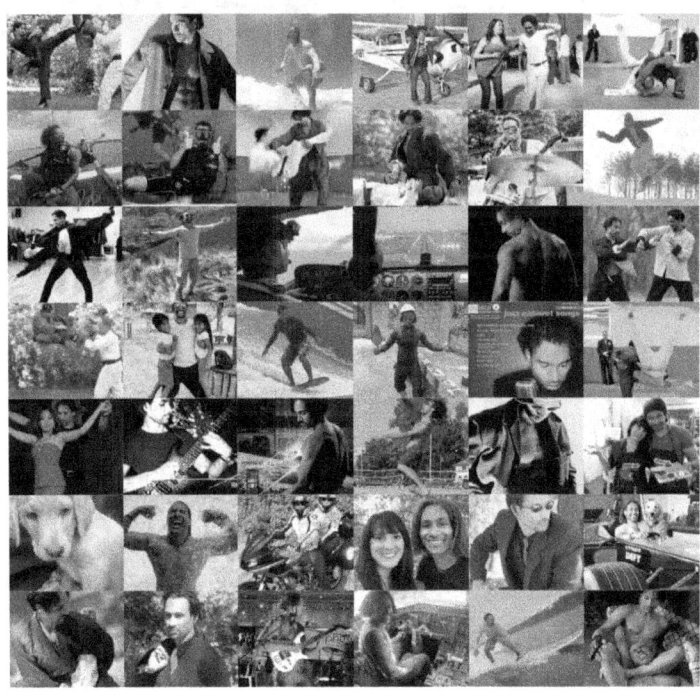

Scan & Follow/Like/Subscribe: Facebook, Instagram, YouTube: @senseipublishing

Scan using your phone/iPad camera for Social Media
Visit us at www.senseipublishing.com and sign up for our newsletter to learn more about our exciting books and to experience our FREE Guided Meditations for Kids & Adults.

www.ingramcontent.com/pod-product-compliance
Lightning Source LLC
Chambersburg PA
CBHW072117070526
44585CB00016B/1486